Josué NTUMBA NTUMBA

Diagnosis and assessment of tuberculosis

Josué NTUMBA NTUMBA

Diagnosis and assessment of tuberculosis

by the Zhiel Nielsen staining method in Lubumbashi

ScienciaScripts

Imprint

Cover image: www.ingimage.com

This book is a translation from the original published under ISBN 978-620-6-73016-3.

Publisher:
Sciencia Scripts
is a trademark of
Dodo Books Indian Ocean Ltd. and OmniScriptum S.R.L publishing group

120 High Road, East Finchley, London, N2 9ED, United Kingdom
Str. Armeneasca 28/1, office 1, Chisinau MD-2012, Republic of Moldova, Europe
Managing Directors: Ieva Konstantinova, Victoria Ursu
info@omniscriptum.com

Printed at: see last page
ISBN: 978-620-8-62433-0

EPIGRAPH

" Looking up, learning beyond; seeking to rise ever higher "

Louis Pasteur

" Yes, goodness and mercy will follow me all the days of my life, and I will dwell in the house of the Lord to the end of my days."

Psalm 23:6

DEDICATION

To the Lord of hosts, Almighty God, my all in all, the condition of my existence, for protecting and supporting me through all the trials have encountered throughout my intellectual training.

ACKNOWLEDGEMENTS

This work, as imperfect as any human work, is the culmination of long years of toil, endurance and perseverance in pursuit of this reward. It is the fruit of considerable effort, made with the aim of honourably obtaining a well-deserved reward.

I would like to express my deepest thanks to : To Professor Dr Christophe NYEMBO MUKENA who, despite his many other daily tasks, agreed to give up some of his time to supervise us with ardour, responsibility and love in the completion of this work.

To Dr Sosthene Kalwaba, for co-directing this work, in addition to his many professional occupations.To the teaching staff and all the lecturers at the Faculty of Medicine at the University of Lubumbashi, who have contributed to my training and to whom I express my gratitude.

To my parents : Caleb MBIYE NTUMBA and Esther MBIYE BAMANA, for their love, support, trust, education marked by discipline, respect and humility, and for their prayers.
May the Most High give them long life, and grant me the grace to honour them.

To my late grandparents : Dr Léopold MBIYE LUKUSA KONDO and Hélène MBUYI KAZADI, whose simplicity, loyalty, honesty and dedication make them role models for the family. Beyond their passing, this work is truly an honour and a source of pride for them.

To all my uncles and aunts, and in particular to : Louis TSHIMWANGA, Liliane MBIYE, Bea MBIYE, Colombo MANGALA, Nicole MBIYE to whom I will never find enough words to express my gratitude and deep appreciation for so many sacrifices made on my behalf.To all my brothers and sisters, and in particular to : Mamou MBUYI, Sandra NGOIE, Gédeon MBIYE, Rachel MBIYE, Myriam Mbiye, Dorcas MBIYE, Sarah MBIYE, Isaac MBIYE, Sharon MBIYE, Janine

TSHABENDE, Laurent NSANGWA, Timothée NGINGIDI, Daniel MUBIALA.To my fellow students and friends, including : Aldehyde KAYA, Morgan MAKUSUDI, Dieudonné TAWABA, Tonton TSHIKANGU, Brandy NGIYA, Clément NDUMBI, Nelly SANGWA, Fabrice TSHIBANGU, Diane SAMBWE, Cynthia OTIKE, Léon MUWAKA, Ezéchiel NSOMBE, Pierre KIDASI, Peguy GOMBO, Fely BAKADIPANDA, Erick NGANDU, David ANGA, Danny KAPAPA, Christel NKATA, Alice NTUMBA, Pierre NTUMBA...

To all the other people who are not mentioned by name here, but who are dear to my heart and who, through their love and kindness, have undoubtedly made their contribution. My special thoughts go to my sisters Ruth MBIYE and Rebecca MBIYE, who are no longer with us, and to my uncles Ruben NZUNGU and Emery KALAMBA, to whom I would like to pay tribute.

SUMMARY

The emergence of new infectious diseases and the re-emergence of pathogens that were thought to be under control is a global problem. Today, travel is increasingly easy. Any part of the world can be confronted with the appearance of a new disease or pathogen that can spread under favourable circumstances. Lubumbashi's geographical position, at the crossroads of several cities, makes it more vulnerable to this kind of problem. Tuberculosis is a contagious bacterial infection, the current epidemiological situation of which is alarming in developing countries; on the other hand, it is on the rise again in developed countries, due in particular to acquired immunodeficiency syndrome. With this in mind, we decided to use the ZHIEL NEELSEN staining method to describe the bacilloscopic aspects of tuberculosis observed during an episode in the population of Lubumbashi. We conducted a retrospective descriptive study, from January 2014 to December 2015, on 605 cases of patients admitted to the laboratory department of the Société Nationale des Chemins de Fer du Congo (SNCC) hospital. The sex ratio was 1.8 and the age group most affected was 26 to 56 years, representing 46.5% of patients. The average age of patients was 22 years. We noted that more than three-quarters of patients, i.e. 87.8%, had a negative bacilloscopy. Most of the patients in our study came from the commune of Kampemba (44%). In view of our results, and particularly the weakness observed in control and follow-up, we believe that the emphasis must be placed on educating the population and training healthcare staff in the management of tuberculosis.

GENERAL INTRODUCTION

Tuberculosis is a very old contagious, endemic-epidemic infectious disease, nosological unity and actual cause of which have only been known since the 19th century. In addition to pulmonary tuberculosis, which accounts for 90% of infections caused by mycobacteria of the tuberculosis complex, these bacteria also infect areas outside the lungs, notably the genitals, meninges, lymph nodes, kidneys, bones, miliary cavities, etc. (**Carbonelle et al, 2003; Helari and Vergez, 1993**).

It is essentially transmitted from person to person, and is currently a growing worldwide scourge. It has a high global profile because it is most prevalent in developing countries, which account for 9/10ths of the world's population. As a result, it is now the leading cause of death from communicable diseases (**Pierre et al, 2004**).

The WHO estimates that nearly 2 billion people worldwide are infected with live bacilli that have retained their ability to colonise and spread. Twenty million of them are carriers of active tuberculosis, which means they are colonising and spreading the bacilli. Every year, almost 1.8 million people with tuberculosis die. In addition, 8.8 million new cases of tuberculosis appear every year, of which more than 3 million are considered to be contagious. Among these infected people, the WHO has identified 4 million cases of bacilloscopy-positive pulmonary tuberculosis (**Pierre et al, 2004**). Tuberculosis is a heavy economic burden because, in addition to its uneven geographical distribution, which reveals a higher incidence in Asia, the WHO shows that in developing countries, the disease predominantly affects the most economically active age groups. At present, the unevenness of epidemic situations, exposure to risk factors and anti-tuberculosis strategies mean that there is a clear distinction between :

- low-prevalence countries, generally industrialised, where the main objective may be to eliminate the disease.

o high-prevalence countries, generally developing countries, where the primary objective is to control the disease.

Sub-Saharan Africa, which represents around 11% of the world's population, reported 24% of tuberculosis cases, 26% of which were tuberculosis. contagious pulmonary disease. The estimated incidence of contagious tuberculosis is 62.6 per 100,000 inhabitants on average worldwide; in sub-Saharan Africa, it is 149 per 100,000 inhabitants **(Pierre et al, 2004).**

In the Democratic Republic of Congo (DRC), more than 100,000 cases have been recorded and are being medically monitored; more than 85% of new contagious cases affect the 15 to 54 age group, with a predominance of men **(Harrils et al, 1996).** This age group, it is emphasised, also corresponds to the age at which the transmission of HIV/AIDS is highest. The disease causes 2 or 3 months' absence from work or school, contributing significantly to the fall in productivity in the country and justifying its heavy economic burden. Of the 22 countries most affected by the , the DRC ranks ^{11th}, and 5th in Africa.

At the level of the provincial coordination of the fight against tuberculosis in South Katanga, the incidence of tuberculosis in 2010 was estimated at 0.18% for a population estimated at 3,636,747 inhabitants, and the death rate among new cases of microscopy-positive tuberculosis was estimated at 5% for 3,687 cases recorded during the same year (**2010 Annual Report**).

Diagnosis still relies heavily on sputum microscopy, which is unsuitable for a large proportion of patients. The effectiveness of BCG vaccination is very limited. What's more, the number of cases detected is rising as result of exposure to risk factors that are ignored and neglected.

This is what prompted us to carry out the study on tuberculosis and to set ourselves the following objectives in our work:

☐ General: To describe the biological aspects, using the Ziehl Nielsen staining method, observed during an episode of tuberculosis in the population of Lubumbashi.

☐ **Specific**:

▪ To evaluate the effectiveness of the Ziehl method in the diagnosis and management of tuberculosis.

▪ Carry out a biological assessment of the course of the disease.

▪ to determine the number of cases of tuberculosis with positive and negative baciloscopy at the SNCC hospital.

This is a retrospective cross-sectional study, based on the results of sputum stained using the Ziehl Nielsen method, collected in the laboratory of the SNCC hospital in Lubumbashi.

We divided our work two parts:

- A theoretical section, covering general information on tuberculosis, the pathogen, diagnosis and treatment.
- A practical section, including a description of the research framework, the materials and methods used, a presentation of the results, a discussion and comments, and a conclusion.

Finally, a number of recommendations bring this work to a close.

PART I

THEORETICAL CONSIDERATIONS

CHAPTER I

GENERAL INFORMATION

1. DEFINITION OF TUBERCULOSIS

Tuberculosis is a transmissible and contagious infectious disease caused by a mycobacterium of the tuberculosis complex, corresponding to various germs and principally **Mycobacterium tuberculosis** or Koch's bacillus (**Pierre et al, 2004**).

2. EPIDEMIOLOGY

Tuberculosis is still a widespread disease; 7 million people are infected worldwide, 3/4 of whom live in developing countries. Every year, 3.5 million new contagious cases are recorded, and the number of people infected each year is estimated at between 5 and 8 million. Some 2 to 3 million people still die of tuberculosis every year. With a population of over 65 million, and an estimated incidence of pulmonary tuberculosis of over 150 cases per 100,000, the DRC is one of the 22 most affected countries in the world.According to a WHO report published at the end of 2011, the DRC ranks eleventh out of the 22 countries most affected by tuberculosis in the world, and fifth in Africa. The shortage of medicines and strikes by the medical profession are sometimes at the root of the increase in the rate of the disease, argued a former tuberculosis sufferer (**Pierre et al, 2004**).

3. ETIOLOGY

Tuberculosis is the disease caused by Mycobacterium tuberculosis, isolated by Robert Koch in 1882 (Koch's bacillus: BK). Mycobacterium africanum is a variety sometimes found in West Africa, which is often resistant to thiocetazone. Mycobacterium bovis is responsible for tuberculosis in domestic and wild cattle, and can rarely be transmitted to humans through unpasteurised or unboiled milk. These three species of bacilli are tuberculous mycobacteria and make up the "tuberculosis complex". These bacteria are said to be **acid-alcohol-resistant,** meaning that once stained with fuchsin or a fluorochrome such as auramine or rhodamine, they cannot be discoloured by either acids or alcohol. It is therefore a Tinctorial property which is the basis of Ziehl-Nielsen colouring (**Jean et al, 1992**).

4. PATHOGENY

Tuberculosis is a bacterial disease, contagious mainly by air. It is transmitted from person to person. In exceptional cases, the bacilli can be transmitted to humans via the unsterilised milk of a sick cow. Tuberculosis can affect any tissue in the body. Pulmonary tuberculosis is the most common; extra-pulmonary tuberculosis is rarer. Only pulmonary tuberculosis is contagious **(Nadia and Donald, 1999).**

4.1. SOURCES INFECTION

The tuberculosis bacillus is a non-telluric bacillus whose main reservoir is patients with pulmonary tuberculosis. In fact, such patients often have 'pulmonary caverns' rich in bacilli (100 million bacilli for a cavern around 2 cm in diameter).

The diagnosis of pulmonary tuberculosis is easily made in these patients, as they always present with long-lasting respiratory symptoms: cough and sputum. Diagnosis is straightforward, as the bacilli in their sputum are very numerous (over 5,000 bacilli per millilitre) and can be found on direct microscopic examination of a smear of this sputum. These patients are known as "smear-positive" and are the main source of contagion or transmission of tuberculosis **(Nadia and Donald, 1999).**

4.2. CONTAMINATION AND PRIMARY INFECTION

When a patient suffering from pulmonary tuberculosis speaks, and especially when he coughs or sneezes, he disperses around him an aerosol made up of droplets of muco-purulent bronchial secretions, each of which contains a few bacilli: these are the infecting droplets. The number of infectious droplets released into the atmosphere by a patient is very high when coughing (3,500) or sneezing (1 million). On contact with the air, these droplets dry out on the surface and become very light particles still containing live bacilli, which remain in the air. suspended in the air for some time. In a closed room, droplets can remain suspended in the air for a long time, and bacilli can remain alive for several hours in the dark: these are "infecting particles". Direct sunlight rapidly destroys bacilli, so ventilation and sunlight in rooms where tuberculosis patients live reduce the risk of contamination for people living in contact with them. People living or sleeping close to a person with tuberculosis are exposed inhaling "infecting particles". In a person who has inhaled the "infecting particles", the large particles are deposited on the mucous membrane of the nasopharynx or the tracheobronchial tree and are expelled by the mucociliary purification system. The finest particles, less than one micron in diameter, can penetrate through the bronchioles to the alveoli of a person who is not yet infected. The risk of contagion is greater the closer the contact, because it is linked to the density of bacilli in the air breathed in. This means that a high proportion of children living close to a source of contamination will become infected. All these clinical and immunological phenomena observed after the contamination of a healthy subject constitute primary tuberculosis infection. It confers a certain degree of immunity on the infected individual. In most cases, primary tuberculosis infection is asymptomatic and goes unnoticed. It results in tuberculin conversion: the subject's intradermal tuberculin reaction, which was negative before infection, becomes positive 6 to 12 weeks after the infecting contact. This tuberculin conversion is proof of recent infection and reflects the immunity that has resulted. Infection of a healthy subject with the tuberculosis bacillus, or primary infection, results in the appearance of a delayed hypersensitivity reaction to tuberculin and cell-mediated immunity occurring more than a month after the first infection with Mycobacterium tuberculosis **(Nadia and Donald, 1999).**

4.3. SETTING UP SECONDARY HOUSEHOLDS

Infection generally stops at this stage. But before immunity sets in, bacilli from the initial infectious site or satellite lymph node are transported and disseminated throughout the body by lymphatic and then blood routes. Secondary foci, containing a limited number of bacilli, are thus formed, particularly in the lymph nodes, serosa, meninges, bones, liver, kidney and lung. As soon as there is an immune response, most of these foci heal spontaneously. However, some bacilli remain quiescent in secondary foci for months or years. Different causes likely to reduce the body's defences can lead to reactivation of the bacilli and their multiplication in one of these foci. This reactivation is the cause of all extra-pulmonary tuberculosis and some pulmonary tuberculosis, which is due to endogenous reactivation. The extra-pulmonary tuberculosis that occurs and the rare forms of generalised tuberculosis (miliary with or without meningitis) do not constitute new sources of infection **(Nadia and Donald, 1999).**

4.4. PULMONARY TUBERCULOSIS DISEASE

Pulmonary tuberculosis occurs in a previously infected person in the event of massive contagion and/or immune deficiency by one of the following three mechanisms:

o or, rarely, by progressive worsening of the initial focus of the primary infection;

- or by endogenous reactivation of bacilli that remained quiescent after primary infection. In the absence of treatment and immunodeficiency, this risk has been estimated at 5 to 10% in the 3 to 5 years following primary infection, and 5% for the rest of life;
- or by exogenous reinfection: the bacilli causing this tuberculosis come from a new contamination. The distribution of the different mechanisms depends on the density of sources of infection in a community: in countries with a high number of sources of infection, exogenous reinfection is frequent; in countries with fewer sources of infection, endogenous reactivation is the most important mechanism for the occurrence of post-primary tuberculosis.

Whatever the mechanism, the immune response secondary to the primary infection is insufficient to prevent the multiplication of bacilli in a focus which becomes the site of caseous necrosis. Its liquefaction and caseous evacuation via the bronchi lead to the formation of a cavity in the lung: the pulmonary cavern **(Nadia and Donald, 1999)**.

4.5. EVOLUTION OF THE DISEASE AND TRANSMISSION CYCLE

The fact that pulmonary tuberculosis develops without any treatment explains the perpetuation of the disease: 30% of patients recover spontaneously thanks to treatment with Patients with extra-pulmonary tuberculosis will either die or recover spontaneously, often at the cost of significant after-effects that can be disabling (**Nadia and Donald, 1999).**

5. PATHOPHYSIOLOGY

During primary infection with the tubercle bacillus, the immune defences of the immunocompetent host are able to contain the infection and prevent the disease breaking out in the majority of cases. However, in 5 to 10% of cases, the infection is reactivated, leading to active tuberculosis and a contagious state. The reasons for this reactivation may be multiple and are probably not all known. Infection with M. tuberculosis begins with the inhalation of airborne droplets containing a few bacilli. In the lungs, the mycobacteria are phagocytised by alveolar macrophages. The local pro-inflammatory response that then takes place leads to the recruitment of mononuclear cells from the surrounding blood vessels, which form a structure surrounding the infected macrophage, the granuloma. The infection is then contained, with M. tuberculosis confined within these structures, but not eradicated. A balance is established between the survival of the mycobacterium and the host's immune defences, which may last host's entire life. When the infection is reactivated, caseous lesions form in the granuloma, in which the bacteria actively replicate. When the cavitation reaches the lumen of the alveoli, the patient is contagious and the bacteria can spread other organs.

6. PATHOLOGICAL ANATOMY

We have identified two types of lesion,

6.1. EXUDATIVE LESION:

In this case, the initial reaction is a mild inflammatory one, with infiltration of the tissues by polymorphonuclear cells and monocytes. This lesion may resolve spontaneously, develop into a tubercle or become caseous. Caseation is a necrosis specific to tuberculosis. It reduces tissue to an amorphous, yellowish substance called caseum, which resembles cheese, hence its name. It can leave a residual cavity, fibrosis or calcification.

6.2. PRODUCTIVE LESION:

It consists of a tuber, the granulation tissue, which has a characteristic appearance. It is composed of epithelioid cells, which may fuse to form the rounded giant cells of Langhans, containing several nuclei arranged around the periphery. The tuber may become caseous, fibrosed or calcified (**Fattorusso and Ritter, 2006**).

7. DIAGNOSIS OF TUBERCULOSIS

The onset is usually gradual, with symptoms developing over a few weeks:

- The functional signs are not specific and may suggest any other respiratory condition: cough and sputum, sometimes accompanied by chest pain and/or dyspnoea. More rarely, haemoptysis occurs, a more alarming sign which leads the patient to seek immediate medical attention (**Nadia and Donald, 1999).**
- General signs include fever, especially in the evening, profuse night sweats, anorexia and asthenia. These signs are not very specific; it is their persistence, accompanied by a marked loss of weight, that worries the patient.

The most frequent symptoms can be grouped under the following headings following:

- 3A: asthenia, weight loss and anorexia.

- 3 T: temperature, cough and perspiration (**Donald et al, 2000**).

In this part of study, we will look at the diagnosis of tuberculosis on the basis of clinical and topographical forms.

7.1. CLINICAL FORMS :

Here we look at primary tuberculosis, granular tuberculosis and chronic pulmonary tuberculosis.

7.1.1. Primary tuberculosis infection (primary TBC)

This is the totality of the clinical, humoral and anatomical manifestations of an organism that comes into contact with the tubercle bacillus for the first time, usually by airborne transmission (**Harrils et al, 1996).**

It is characterised by the following forms:

- **The latent form** is asymptomatic and the chest X-ray is normal.
- **The overt form**: this corresponds to a flu-like syndrome, a history of contagion and the TST (Toxoid Reaction Test) is often positive. A chest X-ray may show a primary complex of adenopathy (rounded opacity), which may be seen in the paratracheal, hilar or bronchial tubes (in this case called inoculation chancre).

7.1.2. Tubercular granule (miliary TBC)

This is the massive irruption of BK (Koch's bacillus) into the bloodstream, affecting the lungs alone and/or other organs (eye, hepatosplenomegaly, etc.). It is in fact a form of tuberculosis with haematogenous dissemination, often acute, characterised by the presence of small nodules spread throughout all the organs. Miliary tuberculosis is characterised by the presence of 3T and 3A, plus chest pain, haemoptysis and variable dyspnoea (usually severe). A chest X-ray shows miliary tuberculosis, i.e. micronodular opacities less than or equal to 3mm in diameter, scattered throughout the lung parenchyma in both lung fields.

The beginning, :

- or insidious: with asthenia, headaches and small febrile attacks.
- or acute: with shivering and a temperature peak of 40 C.°

An unexplained, irregular fever may be observed during state period, oscillating.

7.1.3. Pulmonary phthisis (chronic pulmonary TBC)

In addition to 3A and 3T, we have: chest pain, haemoptysis, variable dyspnoea and the chest X-ray may show nodules at the lung apices, bullous infiltrates at the apices, tubercular caverns (clarity delimited by a fibrous shell which is radio-opaque).

7.2. TOPOGRAPHIC SHAPES

Here, we will review the different localisations and their specific manifestations throughout the body, dividing them into two groups: pulmonary tuberculosis and extra-pulmonary tuberculosis.

7.2.1. Pulmonary tuberculosis

Since pulmonary tuberculosis often causes very few symptoms, the patient may deny any symptoms other than "not feeling well", even when a chest X-ray shows an obvious abnormality (**Nadia and Donald, 1999**).

Cough is the most common symptom, but it can be attributed to smoking, or to influenza that has occurred several weeks previously. Initially, it produces very little green or yellow mucus, and usually occurs in the morning on rising, but becomes more productive as the disease progresses.

Dyspnoea may be the result of a spontaneous pneumothorax or extensive pleural effusion caused by an inflammatory reaction, with a superficial granuloma. Although the latter can occur at any stage of the disease, it is generally suggestive of recent infection (primary progressive TB) in young adults.

Haemoptysis is not usually seen in the early stages of tuberculosis.
Hilar adenopathy, the most common characteristic sign in children, consists of lymphatic drainage from a small lesion, usually found in the well-ventilated segments of the lung (middle and lower lobes), which are more likely to harbour most inhaled micro-organisms.

Pleural tuberculosis develops when a small subpleural lung lesion ruptures and spills caseous debris into the pleural cavity. The most common type The most common is a serous effusion containing very few micro-organisms, resulting from the rupture of a pustule-sized primary tuberculosis lesion. Generally, no air leakage occurs, and the effusion frequently disappears spontaneously within a few weeks. However, it can progress to pulmonary tuberculosis and even spread to other organs.

Tuberculous empyema with or without a bronchopleural fistula is caused by more extensive contamination of the pleural cavity resulting from the rupture of an extensive tuberculous lesion. This breach allows air to escape, collapsing the lungs. In all cases, rapid drainage of the pus and the start of polytherapy are necessary.

7.2.2. Extra-pulmonary tuberculosis

Such distant tuberculous lesions can be considered as metastases from the original lung site, comparable to metastases from a primary neoplasia. In the past, tuberculosis of the tonsils, lymph nodes, abdominal organs, bones and joints was usually caused by ingestion of milk contaminated with Mycobacterium bovis. These infections have been completely eradicated in industrialised countries, thanks to the slaughter of cattle with a positive skin test and the pasteurisation of all milk. Nowadays, organs other than the lung can be infected during the course of a recent tuberculosis infection. Stable infection of a distant site by the micro-organism depends on many factors; some micro-organisms succeed, most do not. Of those that do succeed, many are unable to initiate an evolving lesion and become dormant. Thus, at the site where they are seeded, they may produce an active lesion later, when other diseases are present or defence reactions are diminished (e.g. during HIV infection or old age). The presence of HIV infection greatly increases the likelihood of bacilliemia being associated with what would otherwise be a self-limiting primary tuberculosis. Consequently, a high percentage of TB lesions in HIV-infected individuals are extra-pulmonary, with pulmonary involvement being rarer (**Nadia and Donald, 1999**).

7.3. LABORATORY TESTS

7.3.1. Bacteriology

7.3.1. . Direct diagnosis

The bacillus is identified by microscopic examination and by culture. In our study, however, we will focus more on microscopy.

Whenever tuberculosis is suspected, three sputum samples should be taken for microscopic examination. If possible, they should be collected within 24 hours, as follows:

First sample: during the first interview, a sputum sample is collected on the spot, after the subject has coughed and cleared his throat, under the supervision of a member of staff, in a well-ventilated area;

Second sample: the patient is given a spittoon to collect a morning sample (early morning sputum) before the second interview, which must take place the following working day;

Third sample: at the second interview, the patient brings the sputum collected in the morning and a new sputum sample is collected on site. If the first sample taken on site is positive and the patient not return for the second interview, he or she must be sought out immediately in order to prevent worsening of the condition and spread of the bacilli in the community. A first positive bacilloscopy must always be confirmed by a second positive examination. Any patient with only one positive sputum examination should be examined by a doctor or senior health technician. With three consecutive sputum specimens taken on awakening, it has been shown on numerous occasions that, of those that prove positive, around 80% are positive on the first examination, 15% on the second and 5% on the third. Examination of sputum produced on waking is more likely to be positive than that collected on the spot. This is why the benefit of the third test taken on site is low. Consequently, if the laboratory workload is too heavy, it may be more reasonable to routinely examine only 2 specimens instead of 3. In this case, if it is thought that a patient needs to be put on treatment, even if the 2 examinations are negative, a third specimen will be examined. Before starting treatment, the doctor or technician responsible will see all patients in whom tuberculosis has been suspected but whose sputum tests are negative. He or she may wish to proceed as follows to determine whether or not the patient has tuberculosis: where it is possible to take chest X-rays, if the X-ray shows images compatible with a pulmonary infection, non-specific treatment with broad-spectrum antibiotics may be administered; if the patient's symptoms persist after antibiotic treatment has ended, a second series of three microscopic sputum examinations may be carried out; if these are still negative, the person in charge may decide to administer anti-tuberculosis treatment to the patient. If this is the case, it is recorded as a case of smear-negative pulmonary tuberculosis (**Jean et al, 1992**).

The Ziehl Neelsen hot colouring technique.

The smear is covered with phenol fuchsin and then heated to stain. The smear is then decoloured successively with sulphuric acid and alcohol, and the entire smear must be almost completely decoloured, then recoloured with methylene blue. The bacillus is coloured red by fuchsin and this colouration is resistant to acid and alcohol, hence the name Bacillus Acido Alcoolo Resistant or BAAR (**Jean et al, 1992**).

Practically :

Blade identification

- Take a new slide and use the diamond marker to engrave the sputum identification number on one end of the slide, using the list provided with the samples.
- Prepare one slide for each sample (no more than 10 to 12 sputum samples at a

time).

Smear preparation

- Take each blade by the part where the number is engraved, and place it astride a blade support, with the engraved part facing you.
- Take the spittoon corresponding to the number of the blade, open it and place the spittoon on the right of the blade holder, with its lid next to it.
- Place the metal handle over a red-hot flame and leave to cool.
- Take a sample of sputum, choosing a purulent sample if possible.
- Make as fine a smear as possible measuring 2 cm x 1 cm on the slide
- Place the blade on the dryer
- Flame the metal handle to sterilise it before using another spittoon.
- Prepare the other slides in the same way.

Drying: Leave the smears to air dry for at least 15 minutes (15 to 30 min). Do not use a flame to dry the smear.

Mounting :

- Using forceps, hold each slide by its engraved side, with the smear facing upwards.
- Pass the blade 3 times (in 3 to 5 seconds) through the flame of the Bunsen burner or alcohol lamp.
- Replace the blade on the clean dryer.

Colour

- Place the slides on the slide holder with the smears facing upwards and the edges separated.
- Cover the slides with Ziehl's phenol fuchsin. The fuchsin should be filtered through a paper filter placed in a funnel over the slides.

o Heat under the slides, very gently, until steam is produced, using a pad fitted to the end of a metal rod and soaked in methylated spirits. Under no circumstances should the dye boil or dry out on the slide.

o Leave the hot dye to work for 3 minutes.

o Repeat the dye heating process twice.

Discolouration

▪ Rinse each slide separately tap water until the free dye is removed.

▪ Replace all the slides on the slide holders and cover each slide separately with acid.

▪ Leave for 3 minutes.

▪ Wash with water.

▪ Cover with 70° alcohol.

▪ Leave for 5 minutes.

▪ Rinse again with water.

▪ Blanch a second time acid until all colouring has practically disappeared.

▪ Rinse each slide separately with water.

Counterstain

- Replace the discoloured slides on the slide holders and cover the smears with 0.3% methylene blue for 1 minute.
- Rinse each blade with water and leave to air dry

Expressing results

After Ziehl-Neelsen staining, the number of bacilli present in a patient's sputum is directly related to the degree of contagiousness. For this reason, the result must be expressed quantitatively. The following code, proposed by the UICTMR (International Union Against Tuberculosis on the classification of respiratory tuberculosis), can be used: Code for reading smears stained by the Ziehl-Neelsen method (X100 immersion objective).

NUMBER OF BAAR	CODE USED
No BAAR per 100 fields 1 to	0
9 BAAR per 100 fields	Exact number of BAARs
10 to 99 BAAR per 100 fields	+
1 to 10 BAAR per field More	++
than 10 BAAR per field	+++

For extra-pulmonary tuberculosis, direct microscopic examination is usually negative. The diagnosis may be confirmed by culture of a pathological product or by anatomopathological examination of a biopsy of the affected tissue or organ.

8. COMPLICATIONS AND SEQUELAE OF TUBERCULOSIS

8.1. Local complications :

- Following the persistence of tuberculosis, a pseudocyst may form, which may be complicated by an abscess and possibly aspergillosis.
- The local evolution of the tuberculous lesion is often accompanied by extension to the bronchial tree, with the formation of bronchopneumonia, usually bilateral.
- Pleural involvement is almost constant. Pleural fibrosis evolving into sclerosis, often calcified, may be very marked: post-tuberculous pachy-pleuritis.
- Some neoplasms appear in contact with an old scar of this type: this is scar cancer, generally adenocarcinoma.

In contrast to the extent of all these lesions, adenopathy is much less marked than in primary infection.

8.2. Remote complications :

- Miliaria, multi-organ granulomatous dissemination, is common in cavitary tuberculosis.
- When swallowed, BK resistant to gastric juice can cause lesions in the terminal part of the ileum.

8.3. Tuberculosis sequelae :

Although current treatments for tuberculosis lead to a cure, this is not always achieved without sequelae. What's more, if there are uncertainties about medical treatment, there is the problem of whether certain clinical anomalies are tuberculous or not. Thus, if the tuberculoma does not regress, or only slightly, with medical treatment, other diagnoses must be considered, in particular a tumour in a smoker. The sequelae may include bronchial dystrophy, superinfection by Aspergillus or non-tuberculous mycobacteria, and ventilatory and respiratory insufficiency.

9. TREATMENT OF TUBERCULOSIS

Appropriate treatment of tuberculosis is carried out in two ways (**Donald et al, 2000**): prophylactic treatment and curative treatment.

9.1. Prophylactic treatment

9.1.1. Combating bacilli of human and animal origin

- Promote the education of coughers and the use of new or sterilised spittoons.
- Recommend disinfecting rooms after the patient has left, stables and livestock tools.
- Recommend adequate cooking of meat and pasteurisation of milk.

9.1.2. Field defence

o Combating slums, malnutrition and risky behaviour (alcoholism, smoking, etc.).

o Intensify physical education, outdoor sports and children's work in the mountains.

9.1.3. Child protection

Newborn babies must be separated from the tuberculosis centre as soon as they are born, especially if the mother has tuberculosis. To this end, there are :

- Screening parents with tuberculosis

- The creation of observation crèches and placement centres.

- Vaccination against tuberculosis using the BCG vaccine.

The BCG (Bacille de Calmette et Guérin) vaccine is a live bacterial vaccine, prepared from bovine tuberculosis bacilli attenuated by 230 passages on glycerinated potatoes. The bacilli in the vaccine are therefore alive but have lost their virulence. Introducing these bacilli into the body stimulates the development of immunity, increasing the body's defences without causing disease.In the 2nd stage of childhood, children who are still uninfected should be removed from contaminated areas, monitored in the environments they frequent and contaminated children should be systematically screened by X-ray.

9.1.4. Anti-tuberculosis armament

The basic element is the anti-tuberculosis dispensary for screening people suspected or suffering from tuberculosis. There is also a sanatorium for hospitalising patients with pulmonary tuberculosis that can be cured or improved.

9.1.5. Chemoprophylaxis

More often than not, chemoprophylaxis is actually a treatment for primary infection, aimed at sterilising lesions and preventing the development of active tuberculosis. It is more of a treatment than a prophylaxis in the strict sense. It consists of daily administration of isoniazid for six months, at a dose of 10mg/kg/day for children under 30kg and 5mg/kg/day for children ≥ 30kg and adults.

9.2. Curative treatment

There are five essential anti-tuberculosis drugs. Each has been assigned a letter code:

- ISONIAZIDE (H)
- RIFAMPICIN (R)
- PYRAZINAMIDE (Z)
- STREPTOMYCIN (S)
- ETHAMBUTOL (E)

Some are distributed in combined forms in fixed proportions.

Adult shapes :

a) The RHZE quadruple combination contains 4 molecules in a single tablet: RIFAMPICIN, ISONIAZIDE, PYRAZINAMIDE and ETHAMBUTOL. This The drug is dosed as follows: R= 150 mg, H=75 mg, Z= 400 mg, E= 275 mg

b) The RHZ triple combination is dosed at R= 150 mg, H=75 mg, Z= 400 mg.

c) The double HR combination (HE in the case liver function disorders)

- The HE form is dosed at H= 150 mg and E= 400 mg
- HR is dosed at R= 150 mg and H= 75 mg

d) Simple forms: streptomycin (0.75g and 1g) and ethambutol (400mg) are also used.

There are four categories according to treatment priorities and bacteriological status:

• CATEGORY I :

New cases of microscopy-positive pulmonary tuberculosis and other severe forms of the disease, never treated or treated for less than one month.

This category includes :

- New cases smear-positive TP
- New cases smear-negative PD with extensive parenchymal involvement.
- New cases of extra-pulmonary tuberculosis (in a severe form).
- Severely affected tuberculosis patients with concomitant HIV infection.

• CATEGORYII: reprocessing cases.

These are usually cases of microscopy-positive pulmonary tuberculosis (exceptionally microscopy-negative). 3 distinct groups should be considered: relapse, treatment failure, treatment after interruption.

• CATEGORY III :

New cases of microscopy-negative pulmonary tuberculosis with small lesions and other benign cases of PET and HIV-negative patients

• CATEGORY IV: chronic cases.

These are patients who expectorate tubercle bacilli after an understood and supervised retreatment regime. The majority of these patients have multi-resistant tuberculosis.

TREATMENT REGIME FOR ADULTS

The PATI IV opted for a treatment schedule of 6 months for new cases and 8 months for retreatment cases.

The treatment regimes are :

- CATEGORIES I AND III: 2RHZE/4RH

The diagram has 2 phases:

➢ An initial 2-month phase (intensive phase) consisting of daily administration of the quadruple combination (2RHZE)

➢ A 4-month continuation phase combining rifampicin and isoniazid (4RH), taken daily.

- CATEGORY II: 2SRHZE/1RHZE/5RHE

The treatment regimen comprises 2 phases:

➢ An initial intensive 3-month phase involving daily administration the quadruple combination (RHZE) and streptomycin, but the latter will only be given for 60 days (2SRHZE/1RHZE).

➢ A 5-month continuation phase with the triple combination taken daily under direct supervision (5RHE).

- CATEGORY IV: treatment in specialised centres for 24 months.

➢ Injectables: Streptomycin, Kanamycin, Amikacin, Capreomycin

➢ Oral: Ethionamide, Ethionamide, Cycloserine, PAS, Fluoroquinolone.

PART II

PRACTICAL CONSIDERATIONS

CHAPTER II

DESCRIPTION OF THE TRAINING SITE

1. GEOGRAPHICAL SITUATION

The SNCC Lubumbashi medical complex is located almost in the centre of Lubumbashi in the commune of Kampemba, to the east of the Kasenga road, coming from the city, on the left just after the tunnel, next to the central station, behind the brasserie, in the Tshamilemba health zone.

2. A BRIEF HISTORY OF THE SNCC HOSPITAL

The Complexe Médical de Lubumbashi, commonly known as the SNCC hospital, is located in the city of Lubumbashi, capital of Katanga province in the Democratic Republic of Congo, on the far left of the Kasenga road next to the FINA station and at the exit of the Kampemba tunnel. According to the information provided by the Italian nun of the Catholic congregation "IRMA CANTORELLA" and by Mr MANGI, who was the first driver of the ambulance of the Lubumbashi Medical Complex, it appears that the hospital was built around 1951. It was officially opened in 1953 on the initiative of Dr KANJANGA, who at the time was the departmental doctor.The SNCC clinic was not inaugurated until February 1980. It was built under the reign of Dr BLAMPAIN as medical director of the medical department and Mrs TINDE SALIMA as head nurse. In 1985, large dispensary for operatives was added to staff hospital, along with a number of specialist services and an emergency room. The Lubumbashi/SNCC hospital complex is currently headed by Professor KAKUDJI as Director of the Medical Department, and Dr EPULE AFUMAMBALE as the hospital's Medical Director.

3. CAPACITY

The SNCC hospital currently has 15 departments and around 274 beds divided into 80 rooms and 8 wards:

- Pavilion I: Male internal medicine
- Pavilion II: Paediatrics
- Pavilion III: Women's internal medicine
- Pavilion IV: Emergencies
- Pavilion V: the anti-tuberculosis/HIV centre
- Ward VI: Women's surgery
- Pavilion VII: Male surgery
- Clinical pavilion
- Maternity hospital/gynecology
- Clinical maternity services include:
  - Administration
  - The laboratory
  - The pharmacy
  - Resuscitation
  - Imaging (Radiology)
  - Ophthalmology
  - General services (laundry)
  - The operating theatre
  - Emergency rooms

- The morgue
- The dispensary
- Dermatology
- Dentistry
- ENT
- Physiotherapy

A few details about the LABORATORY service

The laboratory department of the SNCC hospital where we carried out our research comprises 7 sub-departments:

- Molecular biology
- Bacteriology
- The blood bank
- Parasitology
- Serology
- Biochemistry
- Haematology.

4. How it works

The SNCC hospital operates 24 hours a day with 3 duty posts.

1) On-call service from 7.30 a.m. to 1 p.m.
2) Filling service from 1pm to 6pm
3) On-call service from 6 p.m. to 7.30 a.m.

5. HOSPITAL ORGANISATION CHART

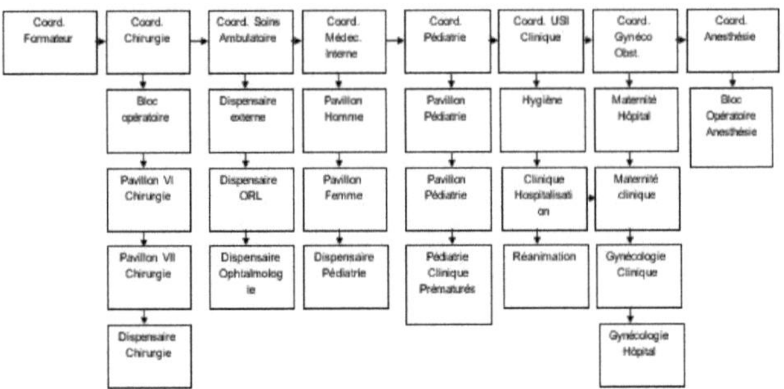

CHAPTER III

MATERIALS AND METHODS

1. TYPE OF STUDY

Our study is retrospective from January 2014 to September 2015, a period of almost two years. We collected data from the SNCC hospital laboratory department.

2. SAMPLING

We identified the trend and prevalence of tuberculosis in the city of Lubumbashi using data and statistics collected from 2014 to 2015 in SNCC hospital laboratory. This was a non-probability convenience sample. We collected 605 cases who were suspected of having tuberculosis and who met the inclusion criteria.

Inclusion criteria: all subjects suspected of having tuberculosis during the study period and all patients whose sputum was collected for examination on suspicion of tuberculosis were included.

Exclusion criteria: All patients with tuberculosis outside our study period were excluded from our sample.

3. VARIABLES STUDIED

Within our study population, we have identified the following characteristic elements:

- The patient's age

- Sex

- Patient origin

- The type of patient

- Paraclinical diagnosis, including the Ziehl test with the different types sputum collected and their bacilloscopic results.

4. STUDY METHOD

We conducted a retrospective descriptive survey based on observation of patient data archives.

5. CONDUCT OF SURVEY

For this study, we retrospectively collated all the files of patients in whom the Ziehl test was performed in the SNCC hospital laboratory.

6. DATA PROCESSING

All the data was collected on pre-established survey forms, the information for which was taken from documents registering the follow-up of tuberculosis patients. The EPI INFO 3.5.1 software package was used group and analyse the data. The data was entered using Microsoft Office Word. 2013

7. DIFFICULTIES ENCOUNTERED

They were numerous, and mainly related to the patients' files. No record was found that showed the clinic leading up to the diagnosis of tuberculosis, but only the diagnosis, category and microscopy result were recorded on the patients' files.

CHAPTERIV

PRESENTATION AND INTERPRETATION OF RESULTS

1. EPIDEMIOLOGICAL DATA

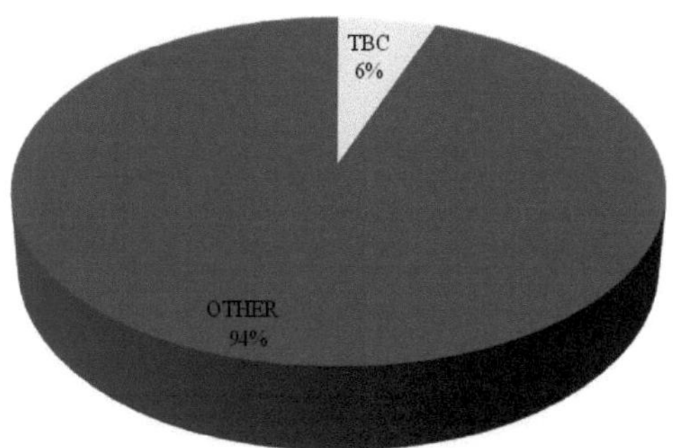

Figure 1: Frequency of BBT from 2014 to 2015

We noted that in this diagram, out of 10146 cases of patients who had consulted the laboratory service during our study period, 605 cases were recorded as tuberculosis, i.e. a prevalence of 6%.

2. AGE OF PATIENTS

Table I: Breakdown of patients by age group

Age group (years)	Workforce	Frequency
Toddlers (24 months-5 years)	2	0,3%
Older children (aged 6 to 12)	14	2,3%
Pubescent (aged 13 to 15)	12	2%
Teenagers (aged 16 to 18)	45	7,4%
Young adults (aged 19 to 25)	143	23,6%
Adults (aged 26 to 56)	281	46,5%
Seniors (aged 57 to 79)	104	17,2%
Older people (over or equal to 80)	4	0,7%
Total	605	100%

The table shows that :

- patients range in age from infants (24 months) to the elderly (80 years or more)
- The average age is 22
- The incidence is 46.5% for adults, 0.3% for small children and 0.7% for the elderly.

3. SEX

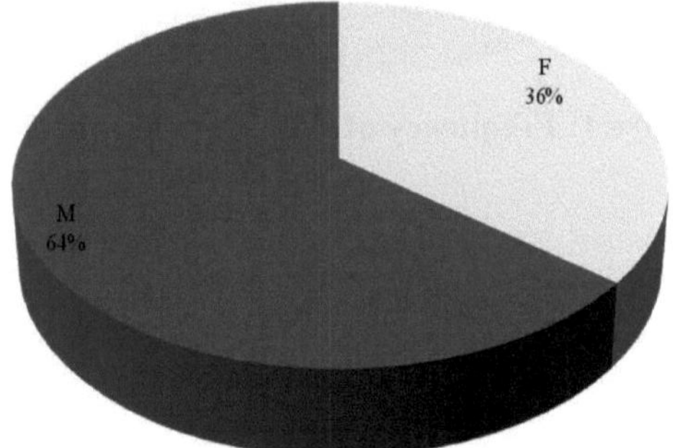

Figure 2: Distribution of cases by gender

In this figure, 64% of cases are male compared with 36% female, with a sex ratio of 1.8 in favour of men.

4. PROVENANCE

Table II: Breakdown of patients by origin (municipality)

Municipality	Workforce	Percentage
APPENDIX	133	22%
OTHER	13	2,2%
KAMALONDO	13	2,2%
KAMPEMBA	266	44%
KATUBA	24	4%
KENYA	18	3%
LUBUMBASHI	82	13,6%
RUASHI	56	9%
Total	605	100,00%

Most of the patients in our study came from the communes of Kampemba (44%) and Annexe (22%).

5. BREAKDOWN OF CASES BY CATEGORY OF PATIENT HAVING UNDERGONE ZIEHL'S TEST

Table III: Breakdown of patients by category

Category	Workforce	Percentage
New cases	382	63,1%
Check at the 2nd month of treatment	77	12,7%
Check at 3rd month of treatment	12	2%
Check at 5th month of treatment	73	12,1%
Check-up at the 6th month of treatment	53	8,8%
Control at the 8th month of treatment	5	0,8%
Other (relapses, restatements)	3	0,5%
Total	605	100%

This table showed that the majority of patients who underwent ZIEHL were new cases, with a frequency of 63.1%. Control at the eighth month of treatment accounted for 0.8% of the total.

6. DISTRIBUTION OF PATIENTS ACCORDING TO BACILLARY LOAD

Table IV: Distribution of patients according to CRACHAT1

Bacillary load	Workforce	Percentage
No BAAR for 100 fields	523	86,45%
Exact number of BAARs less than 10	7	1,16%
10-99 BAAR per 100 fields	17	2,81%
1-10 BAAR per field	3	0,50%
More than 10 BAAR per field	55	9,09%
Total	605	100,00%

This table shows that the majority of patients (86.5%) had no BAARs in their sputum.

Table V: Distribution of patients according to CRACHAT2

Bacillary load	Workforce	Percentage
No BAAR for 100 fields	526	86,9%
Exact number of BAARs less than 10	6	1%
10-99 BAAR per 100 fields	21	3,5%
1-10 BAAR per field	3	0,5%
More than 10 BAAR per field	49	8,1%
Total	605	100,00%

In this table, we note that 86.9% of cases have no BAARs in their sputum, followed directly by the group of patients with more than 10 BAARs per field, with 8.1% of cases.

Table VI: Distribution of patients according to CRACHAT3

Bacillary load	Workforce	Percentage
No BAAR for 100 fields	530	87,6%
Exact number of BAARs less than 10	4	0,7%
10-99 BAAR per 100 fields	21	3,5%
1-10 BAAR per field	2	0,3%
More than 10 BAAR per field	48	7,9%
Total	605	100,00%

The lowest result in the table showed that out of the total number of patients, two had between 1 and 10 BAARs per field, i.e. 0.3%; on the other hand, the majority of patients had no BAARs in the sputum, i.e. 87.6%.

Table VII:Distribution according to all bacillary loads

Bacillary load	Workforce	Percentage
No BAAR for 100 fields	1579	87%
Exact number of BAARs less than 10	17	0,9%
10-99 BAAR per 100 fields	59	3,3%
1-10 BAAR per field	8	0,4%
More than 10 BAAR per field	152	8,4%
Total	1815	100%

In this table, we noted that the majority of cases had a negative bacillary load in the sputum, i.e. 87%, followed directly by the group with more than 10 BAAR per field, i.e. 8.4%.

7. DISTRIBUTION OF PATIENTS ACCORDING TO BACILLARY LOAD IN SPUTUM

Table VIII: Breakdown of bacillary loads in relation to sputum

Bacillary load	Spit1	Spit2	Spit3	Total
No BAAR for 100 fields	28,8%	29%	29,2%	87%
Exact number of BAARs less than 10	0,4%	0,3%	0,2%	0,9%
10-99 BAAR per 100 fields	0,9%	1,2%	1,2%	3,2%
1-10 BAAR per field	0,2%	0,2%	0,1%	0,4%
More than 10 BAAR per field	3%	2,7%	2,6%	8,4%
Total	33,3%	33,3%	33,3%	100%

This table shows that the bacillary load with no BAARs in the chachats is more represented, with a frequency of 87%, followed by that with more than 10 BAARs per field, i.e. 8.4%.

8. DISTRIBUTION OF CASES BY ORIGIN IN RELATION TO BACILLARY LOAD

Table IX: Provenance in relation to CRACHAT1

Bacillary load	APPENDIX	OTHER	KAMAL	KAMP	KAT	KEN	LUSHI	RWASHI	TOTAL
No BAAR for 100 fields	18,7%	1,8%	1,7%	38,3%	3,6%	2,3%	12,4%	7,6%	86,4%
Exact number of BAARs less than 10	0,2%	0%	0%	1%	0%	0%	0%	0%	1,2%
10-99 BAAR per 100 fields	1,3%	0%	0,2%	0,5%	0%	0%	0,2%	0,7%	2,8%
1-10 BAAR per field	0%	0%	0%	0%	0%	0,2%	0%	0,3%	0,5%
More than 10 BAAR per field	1,8%	0,3%	0,3%	4,1%	0,3%	0,5%	1%	0,7%	9,1%
Total	22%	2,1%	2,1%	44%	4%	3%	13,6%	9,3%	100%

In this table, the highest frequency concerns patients with no BAAR in the sputum, i.e. a frequency of 86.4%; and coming mainly from the commune of KAMPEMBA with a frequency of 38.3%.

Table X: Provenance in relation to CRACHAT2

Bacillary load	APPENDIX	OTHER	KAMAL	KAMP	KAT	KEN	LUSHI	RWASHI	TOTAL
No BAAR for 100 fields	19%	1,8%	1,8%	38,2%	3,6%	2,5%	12,1%	7,9%	87%
Exact number of BAARs less than 10	0,2%	0%	0%	0,7%	0%	0%	0,2%	0%	1%
10-99 BAAR per 100 fields	1%	0%	0%	1,5%	0%	0%	0,5%	0,5%	3,5%
1-10 BAAR per field	0%	0%	0%	0,5%	0%	0%	0%	0%	0,5%
More than 10 BAAR per field	1,8%	0,3%	0,3%	3,1%	0,3%	0,5%	0,8%	0,8%	8,1%
Total	22%	2,2%	2,2%	44%	4%	3%	13,6%	9,3%	100%

The frequency of 1 to 10 BAARs per field is almost non-existent in this table, with the commune of Kampempa having the highest frequency at 0.5%.

Table XI: Provenance in relation to CRACHAT3

Bacillary load	APPENDIX	OTHER	KAMAL	KAMP	KAT	KEN	LUSHI	RWASHI	TOTAL
No BAAR for 100 fields	19%	1,8%	1,7%	39%	3,6 %	2,3 %	12,2 %	7,9%	87,6 %
Exact number of BAARs less than 10	0,2%	0%	0%	0%	0%	0,2 %	0%	0,3%	0,7%
10-99 BAAR per 100 fields	1,2%	0,2%	0%	1%	0,2 %	0%	0,8 %	0,2%	3,5%
1-10 BAAR per field	0%	0%	0%	0,3 %	0%	0%	0%	0%	0,3%
More than 10 BAAR per field	1,7%	0,2%	0,5%	3,6 %	0,2 %	0,5 %	0,5 %	0,8%	7,9%
Total	22%	2,2%	2,2%	44%	4%	3%	13,6 %	9,3%	100 %

In this table, we see that patients from the commune of Kamalondo and those from outside Lubumbashi are the least represented, with a frequency of 2.2% for each category.

Table XII: Provenance in relation to bacillary load

Bacillary load	APPENDIX	OTHER	KAMAL	KAMP	KAT	KEN	LUSHI	RWASHI	TOTAL
No BAAR for 100 fields	19,1%	1,8%	1,7%	38,9%	3,7%	2,4%	12,3%	7,9%	87,9%
Exact number of BAARs less than 10	0,2%	0%	0%	0,6%	0%	0,1%	0,1%	0,1%	0,9%
10-99 BAAR per 100 fields	1,2%	0,1%	0,1%	0,9%	0,1%	0%	0;5%	0,4%	3,1%
1-10 BAAR per field	0%	0%	0%	0,3%	0%	0,1%	0%	0,3%	0,3%
More than 10 BAAR per field	1,8%	0,3%	0,4%	3,7%	0,3%	0,5%	0,8%	0,8%	7,8%
Total	22,2%	2,2%	2,2%	44,4%	4%	3%	12,5%	9,5%	100%

In this table, we note that the municipality of Kampempa has the highest number of bacilloscopy-negative cases, i.e. 38.9%, and also the highest number of cases with a bacillary load of more than 10 BAAR per field, i.e. 3.7%.

9. DISTRIBUTION OF CASES BY SEX RELATION TO BACILLARY LOAD

Table XIII: Gender in relation to CRACHAT1

Bacillary load	M	F	Total
No BAAR for 100 fields	53,6%	32,9%	86,4%
Exact number of BAARs less than 10	1%	0,2%	1,2%
10-99 BAAR per 100 fields	0,2%	1,2%	2,8%
1-10 BAAR per field	0%	0,5%	0,5%
More than 10 BAAR per field	7,6%	1,5%	9,1%
Total	63,8%	36,2%	100%

In this table, negative bacilloscopy showed a frequency of 53.6% for males and 32.9% for females. And 0% for males and 0.5% for females, for bacilloscopy of 1 to 10 BAAR per field.

Table XIV: Gender in relation to CRACHAT2

Bacillary load	M	F	Total
No BAAR for 100 fields	53,6%	33,4%	86,9%
Exact number of BAARs less than 10	0,8%	0,2%	1%
10-99 BAAR per 100 fields	2,5%	1%	3,5%
1-10 BAAR per field	0,3%	0,2%	0,5%
More than 10 BAAR per field	6,6%	1,5%	9,1%
Total	63,8%	36,2%	100%

This table showed a frequency of 2.5% for males and 1% for females for patients with 10 to 99 BAARs per 100 fields in their sputum2.

Table XV: Gender in relation to CRACHAT3

Bacillary load	M	F	Total
No BAAR for 100 fields	54,4%	33,2%	87,6%
Exact number of BAARs less than 10	0,3%	0,3%	0,7%
10-99 BAAR per 100 fields	2,6%	0,8%	3,5%
1-10 BAAR per field	0%	0,3%	0,2%
More than 10 BAAR per field	6,4%	1,5%	7,9%
Total	63,8%	36,2%	100%

In this table, we have a frequency of 0.3% for females and 0% for males for microscopy of 1 to 10 BAARs per field.

CHAPTER V

DISCUSSIONS

1. EPIDEMIOLOGY

In our study, the prevalence of tuberculosis in the SNCC hospital laboratory was 6%. In a study carried out in the Lubumbashi health zone and published by Kakisingi et al.(2014), the prevalence was 0.5%. This prevalence is therefore much lower than ours, and so. Indeed, we only took into consideration cases of patients who requested the SNCC hospital laboratory during the period covered by our study, thus reducing the size of our sample and increasing the prevalence. In addition, the SNCC hospital has a tuberculosis control centre, which diagnoses, monitors and follows up patients with tuberculosis, resulting in an influx of tuberculosis patients to the laboratory. This is probably a reflection of the seriousness of the disease in the Tshamilemba health zone, but the high rate could also be linked to an improved surveillance system.

2. AGE OF PATIENTS

Tuberculosis is a worrying public health problem in sub-Saharan Africa, where it affects a young population. In our series, the average age is 22 years, and the most represented age group is that of adults aged between 26 and 56 years, i.e. 46.5%. Other studies point in the same direction, with an average age of between 20 and 30. This is the case, for example, of a study carried out in Lubumbashi by **Kakisingi et al.** in 2014, as well as another study carried out in Senegal by **Mbatchou et al.** in 2008 and another in the same country by **Nafissatou** in 2000. These results are in line with the literature, which states that tuberculosis is more prevalent in young people (www.bfmtv.com).

3. SEX

The results of our study show that men are more often affected than women (sex ratio = 1.8). Although this ratio is higher than that found by **Lawn** in Ghana **in 1998**, it is close to those usually found in underdeveloped countries (**Kumaresan et al, 1998**). Housework that is less exposed to difficult conditions outside the home has been shown to be a protective factor for women. On the other hand, lifestyle in the face of difficult working conditions in a context of The widespread poverty to which men are exposed makes them much more vulnerable to tuberculosis **(Maria et al. 2008).**

4. COMMUNE OF ORIGIN

In our series, most of the patients concerned by our study came from the commune of Kampemba (56.7%) and the Annexe (22%). This can be explained by the fact that patients' access to the SNCC hospital was certainly facilitated by its proximity, but also by the ease of movement to this hospital, which is also located in the Kampemba commune.

5. BREAKDOWN OF PATIENTS BY CATEGORY

In this study, new cases of pulmonary tuberculosis accounted for 63.1% of all pulmonary tuberculosis cases that visited the laboratory; the other cases were microscopy-negative tuberculosis, relapses, withdrawals after treatment interruption, controls and treatment failures. The same observation was made by **Mbacthou et al (2008).**

We found that the incidence of tuberculosis control decreased over time, from 0.5% at the eighth month to 12% at the second month of control. This could simply mean that there has been a significant reduction in the bacillary load in the lungs, or that we simply haven't had the 'chance' to find any at that point. This work also highlights the long delay between the onset of symptoms and the diagnosis of pulmonary tuberculosis, which undoubtedly explains the impact of the disease on the general state of health and the epidemiological nature of tuberculosis in countries with a high tuberculosis endemic, as is the case in our country, the DRC.

6. DISTRIBUTION OF PATIENTS ACCORDING TO BACILLARY LOAD

In our series, we observed a clear predominance of patients with negative bacilloscopy, i.e. 87%. However, when the bacillary load was positive, it was the majority of cases with more than 10 BAAR per field, i.e. 8.4%. This finding is lower than that of **Bousebha et al in 2006**. This could also be explained by the working conditions, which differ between our study and theirs, because ours is a retrospective study, which could be marred by a certain number of biases resulting from the difficulties we mentioned in collecting our data. In addition, the laboratory examination conditions in our series appear to be outdated compared with those in the aforementioned study.

7. DISTRIBUTION OF CASES BY ORIGIN IN RELATION BACILLARY LOAD

Our study shows that the commune of Kampemba, which is the commune most concerned by our study, more cases with negative bacilloscopy, but also cases with more than 10 BAAR per field. Once again, we can justify this by the fact that the majority of patients resided in this commune, which is close to the institution that served as the setting for our study.

8. DISTRIBUTION OF PATIENTS ACCORDING TO BACILLARY LOAD IN SPUTUM

In our series, it appears that the bacillary load with no BAARs in the sputum is more represented, with a frequency of 87%; followed by that with more than 10 BAARs per field, i.e. 8.4%; in the latter, sputum1 is in the majority with a frequency of 3%, followed by sputum2 2.7% and finally sputum3 2.6%. We believe that in this context, this comes close to what is stated in the literature, in that with three consecutive sputum specimens taken on waking, it has been shown on numerous occasions that, of those that turn out to be positive, around 80% are positive on the first examination, 15% on the second and 5% on the third. This is why it is important to always take all three samples for the examination. It's not always easy to find sputum when you need it for tests, as its appearance is proportional to the course of the disease.

9. DISTRIBUTION OF CASES BY SEX RELATION TO BACILLARY LOAD

In our study, bacilloscopy showed that men were more affected than women in almost all groups, except for sputum level 2, where we noted a non-significant excess for women concerning the bacillary load ranging from 10 to 99 BAAR per 100 fields (1.2% versus 0.2%). We did not find any detailed literature on this. This could once again relate to the lifestyle analysis mentioned in relation to the difficult working conditions, in a context of widespread poverty, experienced men, as opposed to domestic work, which is less exposed to difficult conditions outside the home, and which would be a protective factor for women.

CONCLUSION

This study of tuberculosis in the SNCC hospital in Lubumbashi enabled us to note that :

-the prevalence of this disease is 6%.

-men are the most affected

-adults are more represented than other age

-The majority of patients were new cases, compared to other patient categories.

-The patients concerned were mainly those with negative bacilloscopy, most of whom lived in the commune of Kampemba.

In addition, analysis of the results presented in Table VI shows that the incidence of positive bacilloscopy decreases with each control. This leads us to say that the treatment of patients with anti-tuberculosis drugs, if properly applied and effectively observed, gives good results. We believe that the healthcare system for the management of patients with tuberculosis still needs to be improved throughout this part of the city of Lubumbashi, if we are to have any hope of reducing the morbidity and mortality associated with tuberculosis.

RECOMMENDATION

Overall, these results suggest that prevention and case management efforts must be made to improve tuberculosis control strategies. This involves early detection of contagious cases and appropriate treatment until patients are cured. This strategy could help avoid relapses and prevent the emergence of resistance. At the same time, the chain of transmission of the tuberculosis bacillus would be broken and the sources of contamination dried up. It would also be advisable to improve the quality of care for patients whose treatment has failed, by systematically culturing sputum and performing an antibiotic susceptibility test. Antibiotic susceptibility testing is still very important for monitoring multi-drug resistance, and remains indispensable for adapting the treatment of former tuberculosis patients with antibiotic resistance **(Schwoebel et al., 2000)**.

BIBLIOGRAPHICAL REFERENCES

❑Bercion R, Kuaban C. Initial resistance among tuberculosis patients in Yaoundé, Cameroon in 1995. Int J Tuberc Lung Dis 1997; 1 (2): 110 - 114.

❑Botella Hélène ,Study of zinc and P-type ATPases in the interaction between Mycobacterium tuberculosis and host cells. Medical thesis, Morocco, 2011.

❑Carbonelle B., Dailloux M., Lebrun L., Maugein J. and Pernot C.,2003.Biologie médicale. Mycobacteria, Mycobacteriosis. Cahier de Formation 29:158 p.

❑CheD, Antoine D. Epidemiology of tuberculosis in France in 2008. Med Mal Infect. 2011Jul; 41(7):372-8. PubMed | Google Scholar

❑DialloS.HIV/tuberculosis co-infection at the pointG tuberculosis centre. FMPOS/ NIAID, HIV, clinical trial workshop. Bamako 2003.

❑ Eholie SPetal. Fate of HIV-infected tuberculosis patients in Abidjan (Ivory Coast). Med Mal Infect.1999; 29:697-704. PubMed | Google Scholar.

❑EL Helari N. and Vergez P.,1993. Identification des mycobactéries. 90:5-15.

❑Hochedez P. et al. Lymphnode tuberculosis in patient infected or not with HIV: general characteristics, clinical presentation, microbiological diagnosis and treatment.Pathol. Biol (Paris), 2003; 51 : 496- 502.

❑Kakisingi N et al. Epidemiological and clinical profile of tuberculosis in the health zone of Lubumbashi (DR Congo).Pan African Medical Journal. 2014; 17:70 doi:10.11604/pamj.2014.17.70.2445.

❑Kumaresan JA: Tuberculosis. In: Murray C J L, Lopez A D, eds. The global burden of disease and risk factors in 1990, Geneva WHO 1996.

❑Lawn SD, Afful B, Acheampong JW: Pulmonary tuberculosis: diagnosis delay in Ghanaian adults. Int J Tuberc Lung Dis1998; 2: 635-40.

❑LoembaH. etal.

ImpactduSIDAsurlarecrudescencedelatuberculoseetlaréductiondela

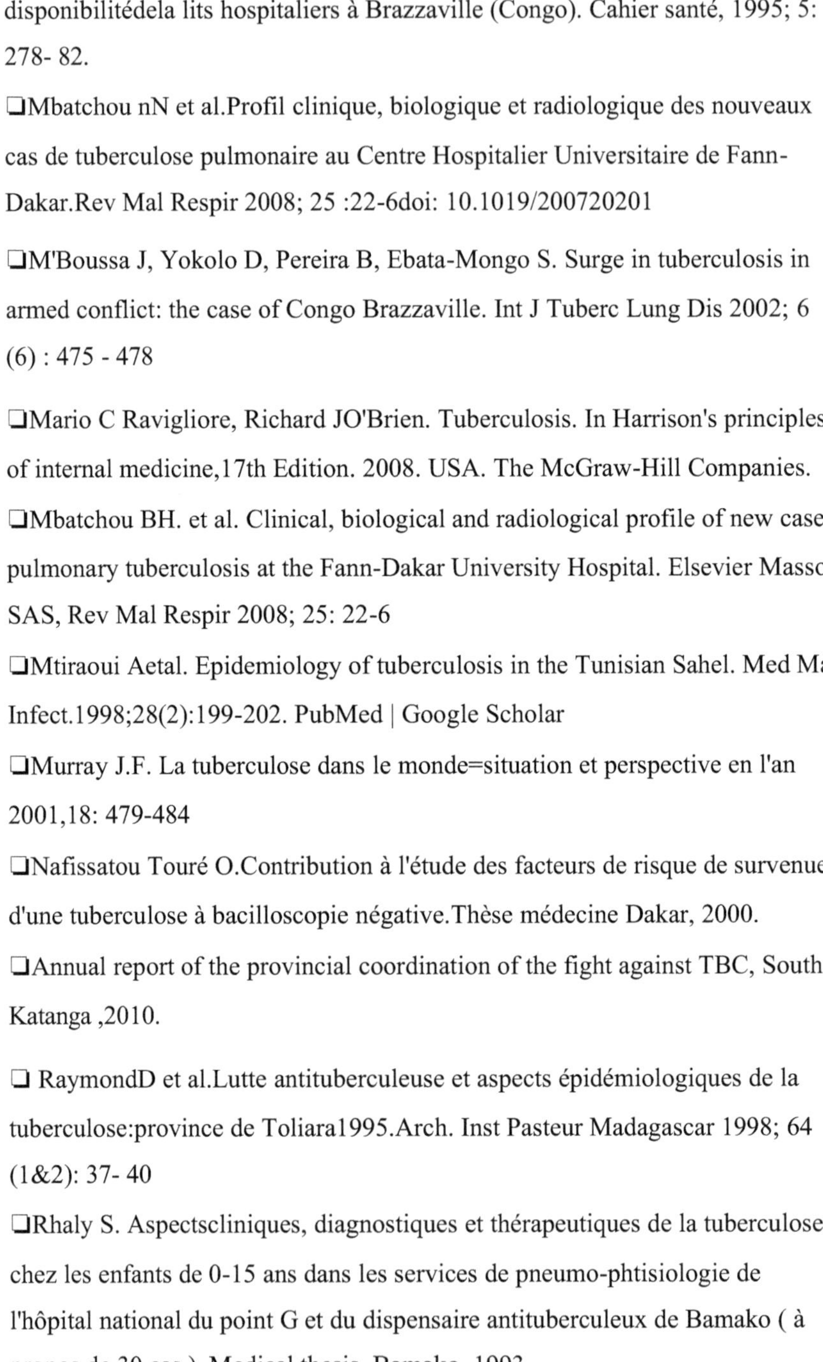

disponibilitédela lits hospitaliers à Brazzaville (Congo). Cahier santé, 1995; 5: 278- 82.

❑Mbatchou nN et al.Profil clinique, biologique et radiologique des nouveaux cas de tuberculose pulmonaire au Centre Hospitalier Universitaire de Fann-Dakar.Rev Mal Respir 2008; 25 :22-6doi: 10.1019/200720201

❑M'Boussa J, Yokolo D, Pereira B, Ebata-Mongo S. Surge in tuberculosis in armed conflict: the case of Congo Brazzaville. Int J Tuberc Lung Dis 2002; 6 (6) : 475 - 478

❑Mario C Ravigliore, Richard JO'Brien. Tuberculosis. In Harrison's principles of internal medicine,17th Edition. 2008. USA. The McGraw-Hill Companies.

❑Mbatchou BH. et al. Clinical, biological and radiological profile of new cases pulmonary tuberculosis at the Fann-Dakar University Hospital. Elsevier Masson SAS, Rev Mal Respir 2008; 25: 22-6

❑Mtiraoui Aetal. Epidemiology of tuberculosis in the Tunisian Sahel. Med Mal Infect.1998;28(2):199-202. PubMed | Google Scholar

❑Murray J.F. La tuberculose dans le monde=situation et perspective en l'an 2001,18: 479-484

❑Nafissatou Touré O.Contribution à l'étude des facteurs de risque de survenue d'une tuberculose à bacilloscopie négative.Thèse médecine Dakar, 2000.

❑Annual report of the provincial coordination of the fight against TBC, South Katanga ,2010.

❑ RaymondD et al.Lutte antituberculeuse et aspects épidémiologiques de la tuberculose:province de Toliara1995.Arch. Inst Pasteur Madagascar 1998; 64 (1&2): 37- 40

❑Rhaly S. Aspectscliniques, diagnostiques et thérapeutiques de la tuberculose chez les enfants de 0-15 ans dans les services de pneumo-phtisiologie de l'hôpital national du point G et du dispensaire antituberculeux de Bamako (à propos de 30 cas). Medical thesis, Bamako, 1993

❑ SchwoebelV., Lambregts C.S.B., Moro M.L, DrobniewskiF., HoffnerS.E., Raviglione M.C.et RiederH.L. on behalf of a working group of the World Health Organisation (WHO) and the International Union Against Tuberculosis and Lung Disease (IUATLD),2000. Surveillance of resistance to anti-tuberculosis drugs: European recommendations. Eurosurveillance 5 :104-6.

❑ www.bfmtv.com / society / tuberculosis-which-is-still-affected-by-the-epidemic- 836086.html

TABLE OF CONTENTS

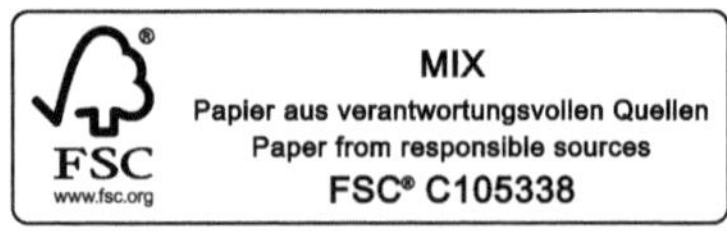

Printed by Books on Demand GmbH, Norderstedt / Germany